101 tips

On Staying Safe At Home with Dementia

Avoid falls, floods, injuries, accidents, doorstep crime and more...

CATHERINE VERNER

Cover Design by Nancy Chrisovergi / Vassil Lakov

Images by Shutterstock courtesy of Foysol Hasan

Editing by Emily Jane Editing

Formatting by Nonon Tech & Design

This book is dedicated to people with dementia and their families.

Table of Contents

About this Book

Globally, dementia is described as a devastating disorder that can dramatically interfere with the health, well-being, and quality of life of not just the person with the diagnosis but with their spouse or primary family carer and the family as a whole.

It is a condition that, historically, has been viewed primarily from a biomedical perspective whereby decline progressively occurs due to the neurodegenerative changes that take place. Failing memory, perception, judgement, and ability to communicate – often tagged as "behavioural" problems - are all emphasised as symptoms of the condition. From this viewpoint, it is readily highlighted that over time, the person with dementia will become increasingly dependent upon others for support and care.

Receiving a new diagnosis of dementia within the family can, therefore, prove to be an upsetting time for everyone. It will bring change and often challenges. One of the main concerns at home will be safety. In fact, it is probably the number one concern. We all strive to ensure our homes are safe, but now it is necessary to take this one stage further as we prepare to take care of a family member with dementia at home.

Caring at home, however, should not be viewed as an insurmountable task. New research is demonstrating that at least some of the negative consequences associated with dementia may be eliminated, eased, or delayed by taking an approach to care that centres around supportive action that continues to promote well-being and sense of self. It is now more widely recognised that the behaviour of people with dementia is not always due to the symptoms of dementia itself but may instead be due to a variety of reasons, such as response to physical pain or feelings of discomfort; over-stimulation from the environment such as loud noises or bright lights; loneliness, boredom or feelings of being socially isolated.

This book adopts this more positive stance by sharing my views, knowledge, and experience of caring for a family member at home with dementia for almost a decade. It provides measures that can be put in place to help avoid accidents and harm and also shares insight into interventions that can work to remove triggers at home that may cause upset or agitation.

Aims of this Book

This book aims to:

1. Provide an easy-to-follow guide on how to address safety and security from a practical perspective.
2. Provide further tips and guidance on household modifications that can help to live well at home with dementia.

Here are some of the areas we'll cover in this book:

- Making the house as safe and secure as possible, both internally and externally.
- Putting in place specific measures to limit falls or accidents.
- Protecting the house from floods and other damage.
- Adapting the house to the needs of the person with dementia positively and encouragingly.
- Creating a living environment that is simpler for the person with dementia to understand and easier for the carer to detect changes in symptoms.

- Creating an environment that offers opportunities to build on ability rather than on restriction.
- Helping promote strategies for safer walking and prevent wandering off and getting lost.
- Providing strategies to enable self-reliant ageing and dementia care.
- Putting measures in place to help stop doorstep crime and other types of fraud.
- Exploring the opportunities offered by assistive technology in living safely and well at home with dementia.

Adapting the environment at home is not a treatment and offers no cure. But many of the symptoms of dementia are subjective; for example, a draught from an open window may cause discomfort. The person may not necessarily know what's wrong – the only indication to the family carer is agitation. But by simply fixing the draught, this agitation would subside. Many potential problems like this can be solved by simple household modifications.

This book includes measures relevant to making the home safe for all older people as well as identifying dementia-specific strategies. A safe care environment is much more than the physical space within the home, so research and background information are provided on the reasons for and importance of each step.

Technology can be an incredibly useful tool that opens up opportunities for people with dementia to live safely at home. So, easy-to-use devices, high-end assistive technology, and everything in-between are all covered.

By the end of this book, you will have the knowledge and tools you need to help make your family member safe and happy at home. You'll discover how life changes at home for someone with dementia, how safety becomes a necessary implication in remaining at home and the measures that can be put in place to address both.

Preface

My mother was diagnosed with combined Alzheimer's Disease/Vascular Dementia in 2011. At the time, she lived alone in a small, two-bedroomed bungalow. We considered various local care homes but it became clear that she wanted to stay in the house she had lived in for nearly 30 years. I felt that option was best for her but as her main family carer I was extremely concerned about her safety.

The years that followed were full of trial and error. We tried different strategies, many resulting in failure, near-disasters, and finding ourselves at the mercy of unscrupulous bogus callers. But we eventually found solutions that worked. As my mother's dementia progressed, measures put in place evolved in line with her increasing difficulty and cognitive decline. My mother remained living contentedly in her own home with support from diagnosis in 2011 until she passed away at home in October 2020.

Having cared at home for a decade, I have extensive practical, hands-on experience of caring for a family member at home from pre-diagnosis through end of life. I returned part-time to study in 2014 and in 2018 I was awarded an MSc in Dementia Studies at the University of Stirling in the

UK, a centre of excellence globally in dementia research and care practice.

This book is one that I wish I had many years ago. I hope that it helps you to not only avoid many of the mistakes and pitfalls we made in the beginning, but to engage with pro-active healthcare, promote self-reliant ageing, and ultimately support your family member with dementia to live safely at home.

Everyone's experience of dementia is different, but I hope that my story will give you a sense of hope. Throughout our journey together, my mother's sense of self remained intact and was reflected n her conversation, humour, and unquestioning certainty that she too was a worthy and equal member of the family at home.

If like us, one of your goals is to help your family member remain living well at home, I hope this book will help you do so entirely or at least for as long as is reasonably possible.

CHAPTER 1

A Shift in Mindset

Finding out that a family member has Alzheimer's disease or any other form of dementia such as Vascular Dementia, Lewy Body Dementia or Frontotemporal Dementia is a life-changing event, not just for the individual but for the whole family.

The majority of people with dementia want to remain in their own home. The problem is, symptoms associated with dementia including impaired memory, difficulty performing familiar tasks, and problems keeping track of things can create challenges at home, especially in terms of safety and security.

As the condition progresses, the possibility of misunderstanding things we take for granted grows. Some of these we know already such as not recognising family members or friends or forgetting details of one's life. However, another common symptom of dementia is a reduced ability to understand the sensory environment. This increased sensitivity to external stimuli can lead to misinterpretation of the environment whereby the person may react to it rather than feel supported by it.

This book aims to help create a home that accommodates these changes – not only from a safety perspective but also on a therapeutic level. One that not only offers safety and security in light of declining cognitive ability but also creates a living space that encourages correct decision-making and enablement – an environment that does not hinder and create barriers but offers the opportunity for safe choices, involvement, feelings of self-esteem, well-being, and ongoing quality of life.

Taking steps to ensure the home is dementia-aware helps appease fears of safety for any family carer while helping to simplify life for the person dealing with their new diagnosis. It provides a foundation to build and work on the more important things that will come to matter in life. It provides a platform from which to move forward more positively and purposefully, nurture remaining ability, and facilitate ongoing connections at an individual and familial level.

Tackling Potential Dangers Lurking at Home

Safety and security are issues in everyone's home, especially the elderly and even more so in the homes of people with dementia. Burns, poisoning, cuts, electrocution, or drowning as well as damage to the house through floods and fires are all areas of potential concern.

Ensuring carbon monoxide, smoke detectors, and fire extinguishers are readily available and regularly inspected is vital. Arranging for flues and gas, electrical or solid fuel heating to be inspected and professionally serviced also reduces the likelihood of household fires and carbon monoxide poisoning.

Falls are a significant cause of emergency hospital admissions in the elderly, often with devastating consequences including prolonged stays in hospital, rapid decline, and increased morbidity. Many people with dementia are unable to return home and are often admitted to a care home after a stay in hospital. Preventing falls and entry into hospital is, therefore, critical for elderly people, particularly those living with a diagnosis of dementia. In fact, it's often on emergency admittance into hospital that many elderly people first receive such a diagnosis.

Falls are not an inevitable outcome of living with dementia. Some symptoms, however, can make people with dementia more at risk due to problems with balance, a decline in gait, visual-spatial problems, delayed reaction, and being on medication that may increase feelings of dizziness or drowsiness.

Sadly, people with dementia living at home, especially those living alone, may become the prey of doorstep crime with many losing life savings. Once recognised as a vulnerable person living at home, they often become repeat victims. Regular victims are added to 'suckers' lists, sold among fraudulent markets. The authorities are often unable to protect these elderly people; the culprits all too aware that their victims prove to be "unreliable" witnesses.

This all sounds very frightening, but don't stress. Simple, practical steps can help to avoid these risks and create a home that is safe and secure from inside hazards and outside predators.

Creating a Therapeutic Environment

For most people, there's no place quite like home. It is more than just a roof over our head; the home represents feelings of familiarity, comfort, and wellbeing – a place where our lives have unfolded.

It's not surprising that the majority of people with dementia want to remain living at home where they hope to stay involved in daily activities, remain engaged in family relationships, and generally just get on with life.

Growing Old at Home

Moving to a new environment such as a residential care home can be a stressful experience, causing fear, irritability, and withdrawal.

Today, many excellent care homes recognise the importance of creating a safe and enabling environment for residents with dementia – the aim being to offer opportunities for stimulation, wellbeing and ongoing functionality.

There is no reason for this not to be the case at home, too.

Maintaining Abilities and Staying Connected

Design on its own will not lead to a successful, caring setting unless appropriate care is available and a positive therapeutic environment is in place. Changes in the house should not only be to safeguard the person against injury but to assist the person to remain engaged in meaningful, everyday life.

Although everyone with dementia is different, there can be a tendency to over-emphasise the deficits associated with dementia, failing to recognise residual strengths and abilities. Taking steps to adapt the home in a positive and encouraging way can help rebalance this.

The aim of making the home dementia-aware is not to restrict the person but to create a safe home where the person can wander, hide things and rummage, free from distressing or harmful situations.

A clean, tidy, warm house that smells nice and has a peaceful and organised feel goes a long way in helping to create a sense of calmness and relaxation.

Understanding Change from the Perspective of Someone with Dementia

People with dementia don't like change. Unfamiliar environments and too much change in the living space can severely challenge someone who is already having problems with recall, working things out, learning, and remembering new things.

The purpose of making the home dementia-friendly is not to make significant changes around the home. Change is primarily for ensuring safety and security, creating an environment that is stress and clutter-free, building on remaining ability, and helping to keep the family connected. It is essential to ensure that changes made are done in a sensitive way, coming from a desire to support the person as opposed to being a reflection of their difficulties. An evolving strategy can be adapted that can match the changing symptoms.

Addressing the Needs of the Family as a Whole

Lack of involvement in daily activities can lead to a loss of sense of self and belonging in family members with dementia, increased stress in the principal family carer, and lack of feelings of connection for everyone at home.

Conditions in the home that support the person with dementia – calmness, gentle stimulation, and involvement – are beneficial for all family members. A home that is dementia-friendly, safe, and secure helps provide a basis to promote ongoing normality and feelings of togetherness for everyone at home.

Moving from Independence to Inter-dependence

Today, the media and government talk a lot about encouraging independent living at home for the elderly.

A diagnosis of Alzheimer's disease or another type of dementia, however, brings change. It is, after all, a condition that affects the brain – the term dementia itself merely a label that applies to the symptoms caused by changes happening in the brain.

Supporting someone with dementia to continue living at home requires a shift in mindset both for the person with dementia and the family carer whereby inter-dependence rather than independence offers a more successful route forward.

Working as Part of a Team

Family carers are naturally very anxious about the safety and increasing vulnerability of the person at home with dementia and are often described as risk-averse. I include myself in that category.

Sadly, the person with dementia is often only too aware that things are changing/have changed for them. Despite this, although an individual may have a diagnosis of dementia, this doesn't necessarily mean that they are incapable of giving their thoughts and preferences on things in the home. My own experience has taught me that the person is still the same underneath – the symptoms of dementia just increasingly muddy the water.

Getting the balance right is important. The job at hand as a family carer is to help put measures in place to maintain the sense of self in the person by making their path and ongoing involvement in family life as easy as possible. A sympathetic, persuasive manner can help encourage the person to accept that changes put in place are necessary to help them to remain living at home for as long as possible.

As time passes, it's important to remain mindful of the increasing vulnerability that the condition brings. A family member with dementia shouldn't feel as if their rights are being taken away although, at the same time, it's important to accept help and recognise it for what it is – a joint effort, a partnership working towards the same desire.

Success comes from knowledge, taking that understanding and working together as a family and applying it in a practical and insightful way. As a family, the only way forward is by working together as a team.

Staying One Step Ahead

The home environment cannot stay stagnant when dealing with a progressive condition. It's important to stay ahead of the game and continue to be observant of any changes. Avoid any crises by taking consistent and ongoing preventative action.

People with mild stage dementia will still be able to live independently; able to function around the home and aware of safety measures to put in place. As time goes on, however, they may be unable to distinguish harmful from safe substances.

Different stages of dementia require separate actions. This book is not divided into stages of dementia because each person's journey is unique. Instead, it includes a mixture of low to high-end measures – some more expensive and intrusive than others. You can judge what is relevant for your family at any given point and how this may change with the progression of time. It can be the case that as soon as one thing is put in place, another requirement raises its head.

There is no single living environment that is ideal for everyone. Some people with dementia will have more abilities and require more freedom whilst some families will have more resources than others. Putting plans in place early in the condition can help allow changes in later stages to come into place with more ease.

No-one says it will be easy, but it certainly helps to have the correct mindset in place from the start. Working together can help ease the transition process from pre to post-diagnosis.

Things have changed. Life has changed. Something you may not have wanted in your life is here. It cannot be ignored and it's here to stay. So like anything in life, it has to be addressed and working together as a team can help pave the way.

It takes time, patience, and effort to carefully plan, build knowledge, and put measures in place to safe-proof the home but in my experience, it is well worth it.

I hope this book helps you find the same.

CHAPTER 2

Addressing Necessary Life Changes

When a new diagnosis of dementia comes into the family, there are a number of initial key areas where change needs to take place. Although this entails the person no longer being able to do things they may previously have enjoyed, it is for their benefit and the family as a whole. With the right information and support these can be put in place.

Smoking

Smoking is not only harmful to our health in general, but if someone with dementia smokes, it can prove to be a cause for concern and a very real fire risk. The person may forget about the cigarette, leave it lit or forget to extinguish or dispose of it carefully. Different situations and solutions will exist for different families. The first course of action, which may solve the problem, is to remove the cigarettes and ashtrays. Once out of sight, the person may forget that they did smoke and therefore, the problem resolves itself. However, it's also about getting a balance right between the person's right to continue to enjoy smoking and no longer being "allowed" to smoke. Ideally, by sitting down and talking to the person, it may be possible to agree that stopping is the best solution. By encouraging the person to quit would be the best decision for their own health, well-being and safety as well as for the peace of mind of the family. From a carer's perspective, the safety of the person is paramount, and if possible to stop, this is the best course of action. If the person has smoked for a long time, on quitting, they may become tense and irritable. A local GP or medical practice may be available to offer advice and support on this.

Alcohol

Enjoying a glass of wine or other alcoholic drinks can be a pleasant experience for most people. It can help people relax and generally chill out. However, in people with dementia, this can add to additional confusion and disorientation. People with dementia may easily forget how much alcohol they have had and continue to drink too much. Alcoholic intake, no matter how much, can increase the risk of stumbling and falling. So, it is important to limit the drinking of alcohol after a diagnosis of dementia. No alcohol at all can prove to be the best way forward. Some people develop dementia that is linked to the excessive intake of alcohol during their life. In this instance, alcohol should be stopped where possible. Another reason for stopping drinking is the mix of alcohol and medication. Keeping alcohol out of reach may prove to be the solution adopted by families. Each family should be able to gauge what is best for them. There are many enjoyable non-alcoholic drinks on the market that can prove to be a good substitute.

Driving

If living in the United Kingdom, anyone with a new diagnosis of dementia must contact the government's Driver and Vehicle Licensing Agency (DVLA). When first given a new diagnosis, this does not immediately mean that the person must give up driving. It is, however, essential to ensure that the person is still able to drive safely. In many cases, people will decide to stop driving themselves or after discussion with their family. In other cases, the person's doctor may advise the person to stop. In some instances, DVLA will revoke the person's driving license.

Being told that you can no longer drive can have a really negative impact on a person with dementia. There is also a big difference between someone making a decision to stop and being told to stop. However, most people, although they know they will have to stop at one time, may find it difficult to identify or accept when that time has arrived. It can often reach a crisis point when the person has a bump or comes home forgetting where they left their car or that they even had one, to begin with.

This loss of independence involved can be different for different people. Some may accept it. Others see it as having a hugely negative impact on their life, especially if taxis are too expensive, public transport is inadequate, or family members not readily available to help out. This can curtail outings, and so it becomes more important that people with dementia can continue to get out and about generally.

Firearms

Owning a gun at home in countries such as the United States can cause huge concerns for the families of people living at home with dementia. When a person is first diagnosed, the discussion should take place regarding the safety of the person with dementia and other family members if any weapons are present in the house. Framing the discussion around the topic of safety may make it easier for the person to accept the potential problem. Options include removing the firearm from the house or locking it safely and unloaded in a basement or another safe place in the house. Discussions around the transfer of ownership may also be necessary. Families in the USA may find it helpful to talk to their attorney about state and federal laws around gun ownership.

CHAPTER 3

Creating a Safe, Secure, and Supportive Living Space

Keeping It Simple

A simple, clutter-free home benefits people with dementia both physically and cognitively. The simpler things are, the easier it will be for the person to navigate the house. Creating clear walkways between rooms and within rooms will also help minimise the risk of falling.

People with dementia often hide things and can spend hours rummaging trying to find them. The simpler and more clutter-free the environment, the easier it will be to find missing items.

As dementia progresses, it may become difficult to use such things as the TV remote, but in the early to moderate stages of dementia, not even being able to find the TV remote can mean missing favourite TV programs or sitting in silence all day if home alone. Reserve easy-to-reach places for essential things that are used daily to keep life simple.

Making It Obvious

A straightforward way to create a home that helps someone living with dementia is to make everything as obvious as possible.

Just as our physical strength decreases with age, our eyes also experience age-related decline. The way we perceive colour also changes with age. This is a significant problem for people with dementia as they may increasingly lose the ability to see and judge depth correctly.

Contrast, vividness, and subtle changes in colour also diminish. Impaired contrast-perception makes it harder to see the edges of objects, mainly when the foreground and background are similar in colour. For example, if a white book is sitting on a white shelf, we will see both. However, for someone with dementia, this may not be the case. Prominent colour contrast can be used to highlight important objects.

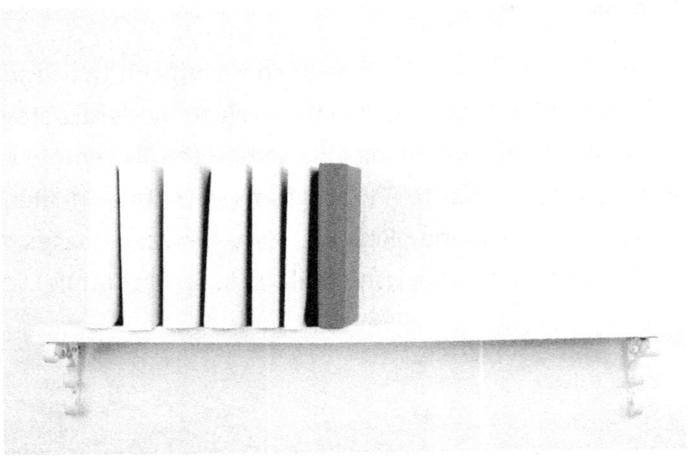

In the same way, a lack of contrast can be used to help objects blend in with the surroundings. An example of this would be making the front door the same colour as the walls to help it blend in and not be a continual visual reminder to leave the house. Alternatively, if we want to make the bathroom stand out, painting the door in a contrasting colour to the surrounding walls will help achieve this.

Lighting it Up

Sight loss is common as people get older, whether through normal ageing of the eye or as the result of eye conditions such as cataracts or macular degeneration. In general, elderly people need twice as much light as the standard recommendation and increasingly find it difficult to adjust to changes in the level of light.

With the brain's ability to make sense of visual signals increasingly diminished, people with dementia are at an even greater disadvantage, resulting in them becoming confused and making mistakes. Poor lighting further hinders this, resulting in increased anxiety and insecurity as to where they are and what surrounds them.

What the eyes see the brain must interpret. As a basic premise, it is important to be able to see the environment clearly to help to even begin to make sense of it. Brighter, even, and consistent lighting throughout the house will help with this. It can help people with dementia to see where they want to go, spaces, rooms, items they need as well as signs and equipment. It will enable the person to manoeuvre the home more easily, allowing them to continually see what's around them and in front of them.

Proper lighting will also eliminate dark spots or areas in the room that appear ominous, confusing, or anxiety-provoking. Clear, bright spaces will help ease the mind and provide a better understanding of the surroundings, leading to increased feelings of safety, contentment, and well-being.

Disturbed sleep is another common problem with the progression of dementia. As the brain declines, it starts to affect the body's natural body clock with night turning into day and vice versa. So anything that can keep the normal wake/sleep cycle intact is helpful.

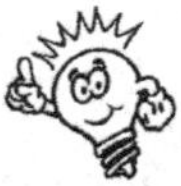

Helpful Tips

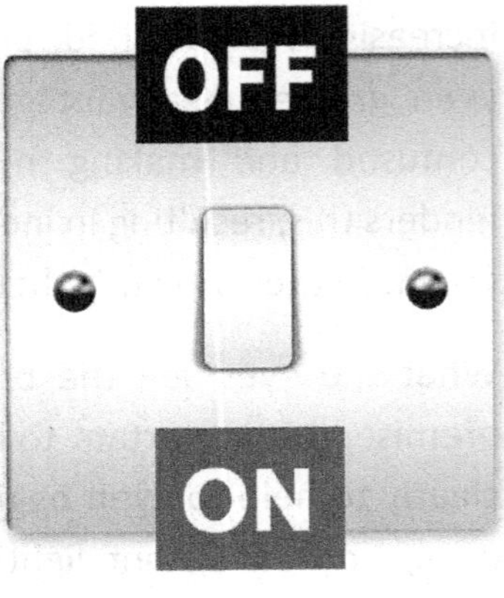

1. Put 'on' and 'off' labels on light switches to act as simple memory prompts. Depending on the stage of dementia, simple easy-to-do instructions such as this can be all that it takes to ensure lights and other household appliances are safely put off when required and at night.

2. Avoid sudden changes in light level that can cast shadows. Instead, make sure all lighting transitions gently between well-lit and less well-lit areas. Adjust glaring lights that may reflect on floors making them look slippery and dangerous.

3. Install nightlights to accommodate visits to the bathroom. Consider nightlights that automatically come on at dusk and switch off at dawn, such as those found at www.alzproducts.co.uk.

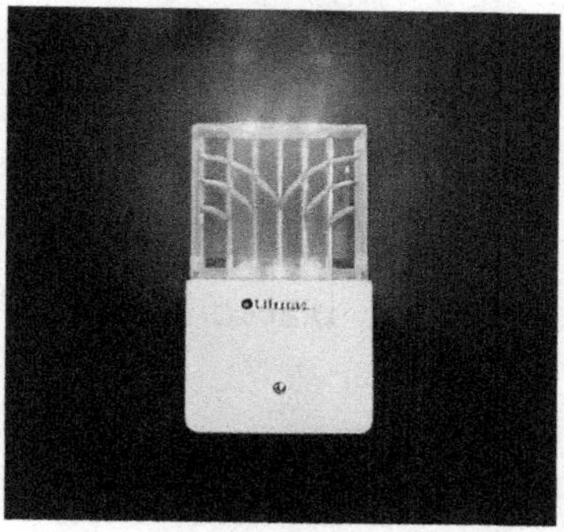

4. Or, install motion sensor lighting that switches on when motion is detected such as those found on www.atdementia.org.uk. Phillips Hue also offers a range of automated lights.

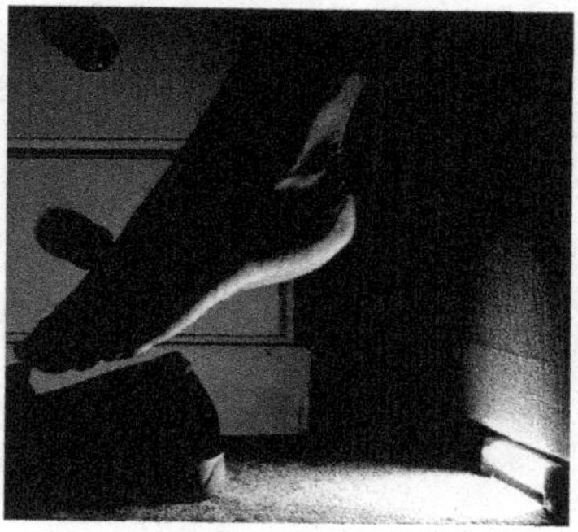

5. Make the most of natural light around the home by opening curtains and pulling up blinds or shutters.

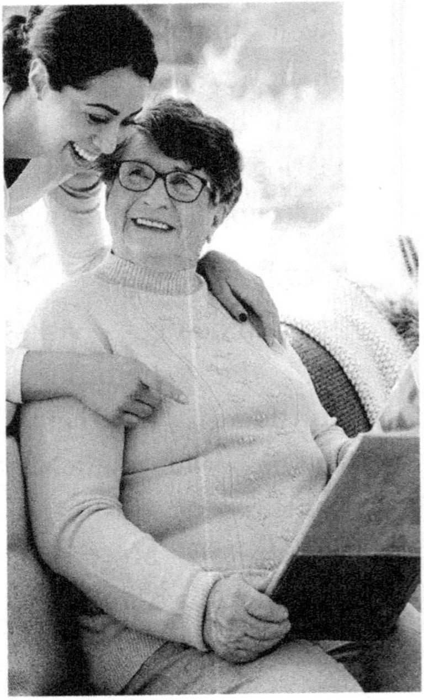

This will also help maintain natural feelings of well-being and help keep day and night more easily identifiable. Ensuring a daily routine is also in place can offer huge benefits in regulating the body's natural clock.

6. Use blackout blinds to block out light at night when sleeping. This can help ensure a good night's sleep and separate night from day. It also helps eliminate shadows of moving trees and branches outside windows at night which can be distressing.
7. Consider the use of light therapy, shown by some studies to help reduce sleep disturbance in dementia.

Keeping It Down

In addition to an increased sensitivity to light, dementia can also bring a reduced tolerance to sound. In fact, an overload of combined sensory stimulation (sight, noise, touch, and smell) can lead to a sudden detrimental change.

Noise that is acceptable to other people in the living space may be distressing for someone with dementia. Strange or loud noises can lead to increased anxiety and agitation; something as simple as a loudly ticking clock can cause fear or upset. If an individual has an impaired capacity to think, anything that can help minimise meaningless noise is valuable.

Someone with dementia may also have difficulty hearing or understanding conversations if there is competing background noise. Having conversations that are face-to-face and free from distracting noise will help, allowing the person to focus on one interaction at a time.

Getting levels of sound correct in the home is essential to allow the person to process not only conversations but the environment around them, too.

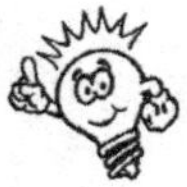

Helpful Tips

8. Strike a balance between blaring TVs and radios and soft relaxing music that provides a pleasant distraction and a feeling of calmness. Music can be a welcome source of solace for many people with dementia. In fact, increasing evidence shows that the ability of people with dementia to connect with music is preserved into the late stages.

9. Songs that are recognised by the person can increase feelings of contentment. At www.playlistforlife.com

you can create personalised playlists that can help tap into hidden memories and foster feelings of joy, happiness, relaxation, and calmness.

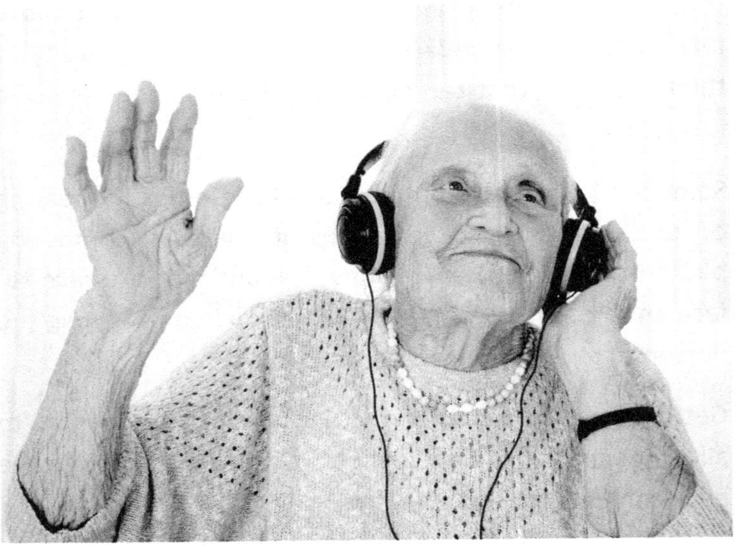

Fittings and Furnishings

Doors, Windows and Keys

It's crucial to ensure the home is secure with all exterior doors having secure safety locks. Attaching a security chain to external doors provides an additional safety measure and fitting a letter-cage over the inside letterbox will help avoid bending to pick up mail that can cause dizziness and falls.

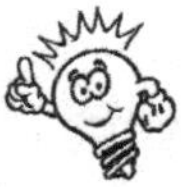

Helpful Tips

10. Patio or standard glass doors can be difficult to see. Put stickers at eye level to make them visible and prevent cuts, bruises, concussion, or worse if walked into by mistake. Ensure sliding windows, especially if you live on an upper floor, are secure and locked if need-be. Locks can be put in place that allow them to be opened enough to let in fresh air but not allow a person to walk through them. Patio doors can be fitted with an alarm as an additional precaution.

11. Install a key-safe on the outside of the house. A key-safe is a secure box which holds a spare key to the home. It can be used in an emergency or by care support staff. There are many different types on the market but good examples can be found at www.keysafe.co.uk.

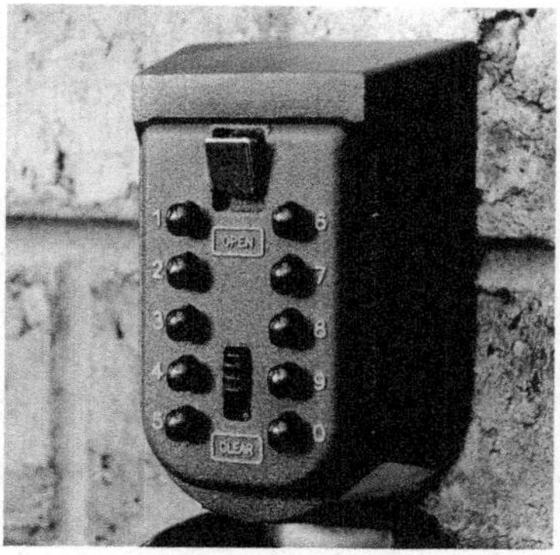

12. Consider removing locks from internal doors to prevent the person from locking themselves inside.

13. Ensure 'no-go' areas such as cellars, attics, basements or other potentially unsafe areas are locked.

Carpets, Rugs, Floorings, and Wallcoverings

Simple measures can be taken to help reduce the risk of falls in the home. To begin with, straightforward things such as sturdy, well-fitting slippers help. Frayed carpets should be removed or repaired and it's advisable to replace slippery linoleum with carpet or non-slip flooring.

Visual 'noise' can lead to agitation and confusion, so consider this when choosing fabric patterns and wall art.

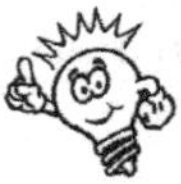

Helpful Tips

14. Remove tripping hazards such as throw rugs, extension cords, and cables to help reduce the risk of tripping and falling.

15. Contrast the wall colour with the floor to make it clear where the floor ends and the wall begins.

16. Avoid shiny tiled, marbled or linoleum floors. The reflection may cause difficulty due to compromised depth perception and judgement, making it difficult to judge when the foot will hit the ground. A shiny, reflective floor may also create a fear of slipping or look like water to be avoided – whether it's a high gloss floor or simply sunlight from a window.

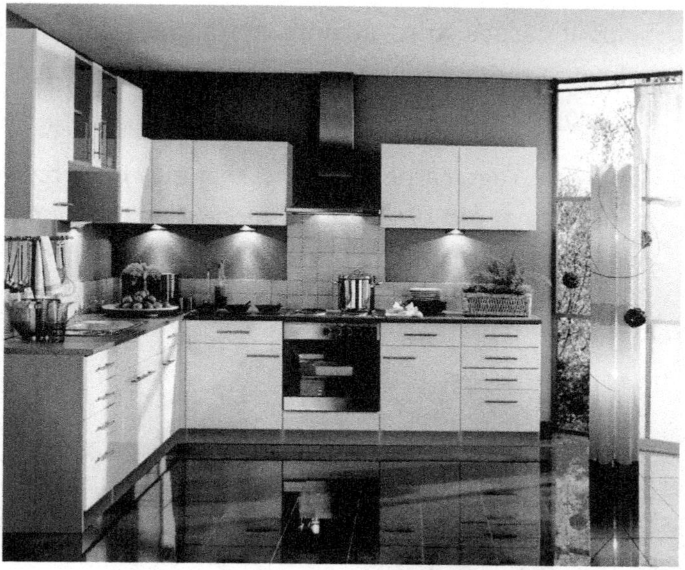

17. Avoid busy wallpaper patterns. These can cause confusion and agitation. Floral designs that look like flowers or bugs may be misinterpreted as real flowers or bugs crawling up the wall.

18. Avoid bold, high-contrast patterns on floors, especially dots, stripes, zigzags, and chequered patterns that may be perceived as steps or moving objects. Also, avoid designs that may be mistaken for something lying on the floor. This could result in the person bending down to pick it up and becoming dizzy or falling.

19. Avoid sharp changes in colour and shade of carpets and rugs between rooms or within rooms as this can often be perceived as a change in floor level or cause concern about stepping into something new. It also

helps if carpet strips at door entrances are a similar colour to the flooring. Ideally, the flooring throughout the property should be the same colour.

20. Avoid dark rugs, carpets, or mats that may be perceived as holes that can't be walked upon, should be jumped over, or stepped around.

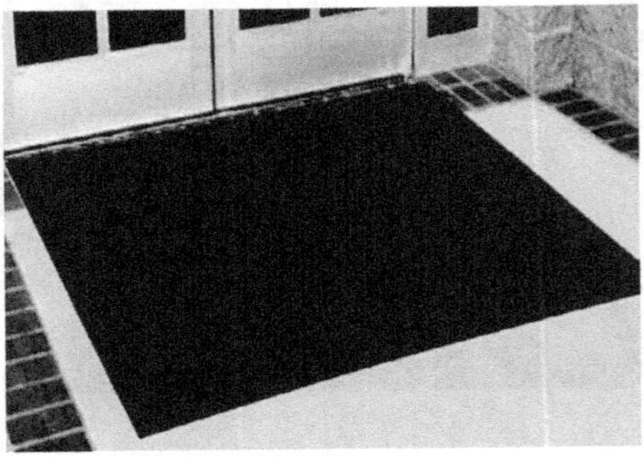

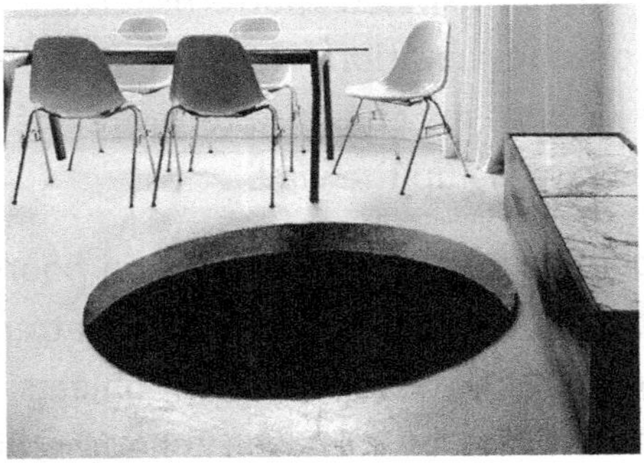

Furniture and Furnishings

Rise and recline chairs greatly help with mobility. Chairs and settees should be comfortable and pressure care seating pads can be used if needed. Good contrast between floor and wall colouring and that of tables, lamps, and chairs can help the latter stand out more.

Helpful Tips

21. Ensure suitable furniture that may be used to lean on and provide support is stable and secure.

22. Consider removing mirrors if they're causing upset. Someone with dementia may become anxious about seeing their reflection. The image may be unrecognisable – a stranger in front of them. Often the image people have of themselves is one of much younger years. A recent image of themselves may be completely unfamiliar and, therefore, cause concern. Whether a momentary glance of someone in a small mirror or the full image of a "stranger" in a full-length mirror, this can cause alarm. A mirror, for example, on a bathroom wall, can give the impression of two doors or two washbasins. Taking steps to eliminate potential misinterpretations will help avoid unnecessary stress and anxiety.

Areas in the House

Stairs and Hallways

An ideal home setting is on one level, such as a bungalow or apartment. But this may not always be possible so certain precautions are necessary. As standard, homes of all frail elderly people should be equipped with handrails for all steps and staircases.

Helpful Tips

23. Remove any distractions like paintings on the walls of staircases that may distract the person when walking up and down the steps.

24. Install clearly visible, coloured, slip-resistant strips and treads on stairs and steps at the edge, a different colour for first and last step is helpful.

Kitchen

Kitchens are so much more than places to prepare food. They provide a social space for family members and friends to unite, communicate, and stay connected. Remaining part of this interaction for as long as possible, even if involved in small activities like folding laundry or setting the table will prove helpful. Making the kitchen as safe, dementia-friendly, and straightforward as possible will help facilitate this. As with the rest of the house, a kitchen that is well organized and not cluttered will help make it easier to find things.

Helpful Tips

25. Add simple DIY signs beside plugs such as 'Switch off at night' (TV, etc.) or 'Do not switch off at night' (telecare, fridge, etc.). These can act as simple reminders.

26. Create a list of contacts including close relatives, friends, next-door neighbours, medical practitioners, as well as gas, electricity, and water suppliers. Include information such as where the stopcock is to turn the water off for emergencies.

27. Items such as medication, alcohol, matches, and sharp objects should be securely locked away. Cleaning liquid such as bleach should be kept out of sight or secured to avoid possible ingestion of harmful chemicals mistaken for drinks.

28. Eating food that is out of date can be a problem. The 'use by' date can be ignored by someone with dementia or too small to read. Continual monitoring of food will help eliminate this. It's also helpful to write when food needs to be used by on a calendar that can be attached to the front of the fridge. A magnetic memo board can also be useful for this. Label all food based on when it's opened. The careful monitoring of food to reduce the risk of salmonella and other types of food poisoning is essential.

29. Ensure all every-day safe objects are easy to see and reach to avoid stretching and losing balance. Use clear containers to allow easy visibility of content such as teabags, coffee, and sugar.

30. Ensure all heated appliances such as the kettle, coffee maker, and iron all have automatic cut-offs and regularly check that they work.

31. A clear, illuminating glass kettle will make it easy to see that water is in the kettle and that it is boiling. Similarly, a glass toaster can make it easier for the person to understand and work with.

32. A lock over the cooker switch will ensure rings have not been left burning. Or items such as electric kettles are not put on a gas ring. Examples of locks can be found at www.securitysafetyproducts.co.uk.

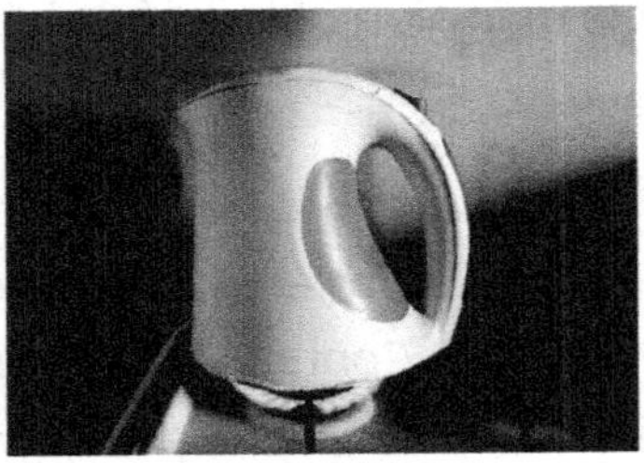

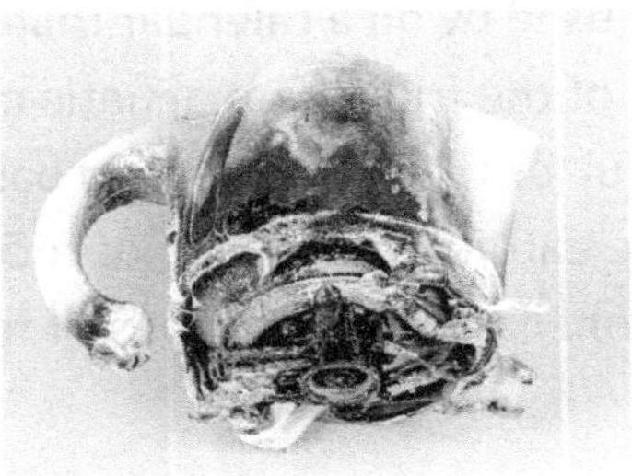

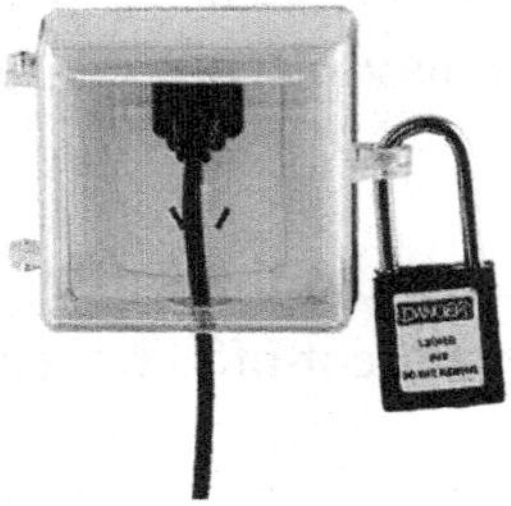

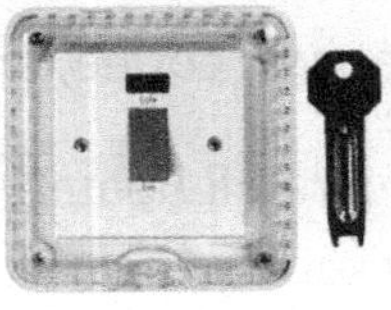

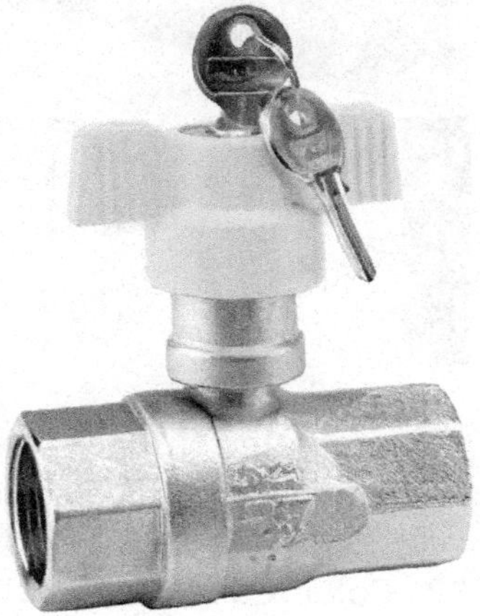

33. Devices such as a locking cooker valve can also be installed by a qualified gas fitter. Some companies offer this service for free. The simple safety device is fitted to existing gas cooker pipe-work. When the valve is locked, the gas supply to the cooker is stopped. This eliminates the risk of the cooker being unintentionally turned on or left on. It can easily be turned back on when the cooker is required.

34. Consider installing the Innohome Stove Alarm above the cooker. It attaches to the cooker hood using magnets or can be fitted to the wall by screws. An alarm is activated if the cooker becomes too hot or when an empty hotplate is left on, alerting carers before a problem arises.

35. Purchase a simple-to-use microwave with a basic instruction panel. You may, however, need to disconnect or remove the microwave based on the stage of dementia to avoid potential accidents.

36. Put photos and/or labels on the front of drawers and cupboards to aid navigation around the kitchen and avoid frustration. A selection of labels can be found at www.alzproducts.co.uk.

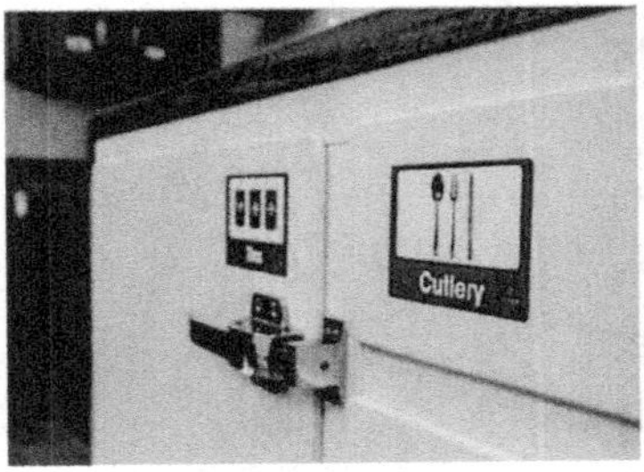

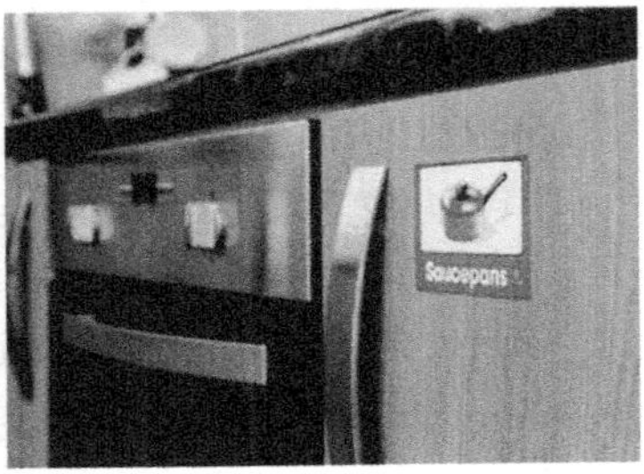

Integrated fridges can be difficult for people with dementia to recognise. Put stickers on the front to help.

37. Coloured rubber mats and/or crockery that contrast with trays or tablecloths help define the edge of plates and dishes and make them more visible.

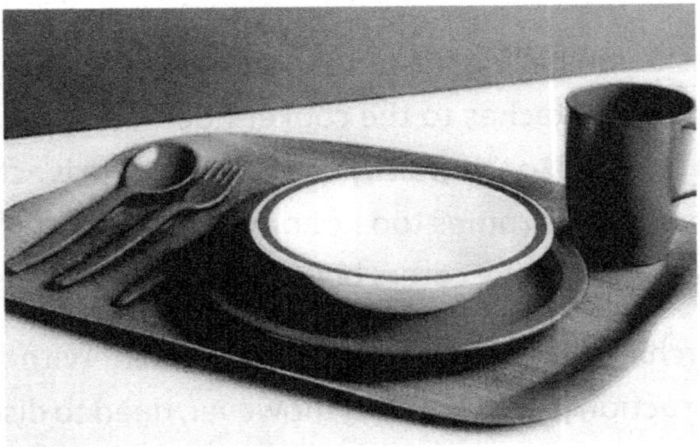

38. Coloured tape on backplates around sockets and switches can help them stand out more easily.

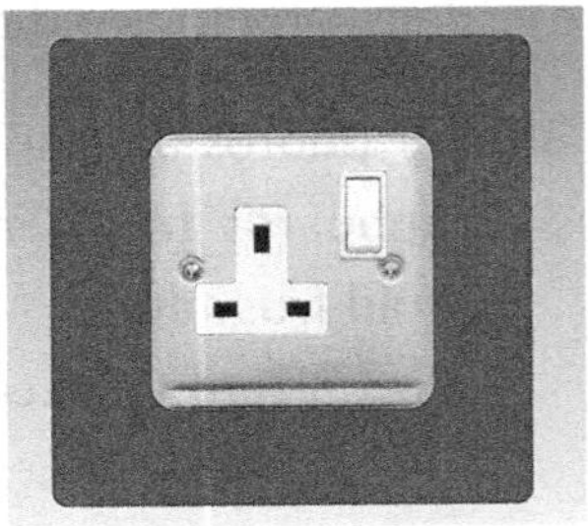

Bathrooms/Shower Rooms

The bathroom can present many challenges for people with dementia. Sensory overload through bright lights, flushing toilets, flowing water, and noisy extractor fans are all things to watch out for.

There is no reason for soft, gentle music not to be part of the daily bathing routine – bathing should be a pleasurable experience. A warm bathroom is also important as cold muscles don't work as well and could increase the risk of a fall. Bath oils and lotions can make a bath or shower slippery so avoid these. Finally, a comfortable chair, if there is room, offers an ideal place to get dry and dressed.

Needing to use the toilet and not being able to find it can cause anxiety, so it's important that the toilet is always easy to find. The ideal set-up is to have an en-suite bathroom or shower room in the bedroom in addition to a downstairs toilet for convenience. With the door left ajar at night, the en-suite toilet would ideally be visible from the head of the bed. Install a nightlight that automatically switches on when the person rises from their bed. Some people may choose to leave the toilet light on during the night, but this may not always be possible or practical.

Helpful Tips for Safer Bathing

39. Remove loose bathroom mats as these are easy to trip over. Make use of non-slip mats on the bottom of the bath or shower to help prevent slips and falls.

40. Consider installing slip-resistant flooring for the whole bathroom floor.

41. Remove glass shelves and replace with wooden curved-edged shelves. Remove all glass or fragile items and replace with plastic, coloured cups and holders.

42. Ensure shower doors are tempered glass and not plate glass and put a sticker on the glass shower door to make it more visible.

43. Install firmly mounted handrails along the wall of the bath/shower and toilet, ensuring any lightweight wall-mounted towel rails or toilet roll holders that may be mistaken for handrails are replaced.

44. Remove or lock away all hazardous items such as medication, mouthwash, and cough syrup.

45. Remove all electrical appliances such as electric razors, hairdryers, or curling tongs from the bathroom that may be dropped in water. Remove items such as plastic razors that can cause injury.

46. Consider changing the door to one that opens out or a bi-fold door. Many people fall behind the door and cannot be reached in an emergency. If possible, modify the door to ensure it can be opened from the outside if locked by mistake by removing the lock or installing a lock that can be opened from the outside.

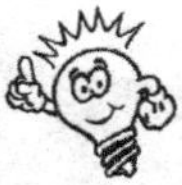

Helpful Tips on Visual Aids

47. Paint the bathroom door a different colour or with a contrasting trim to make it more easily identifiable. Put a photo of a toilet and the word 'toilet' or 'bathroom' on the door as a continual and easy memory jogger. Find inexpensive examples at www.gompels.co.uk

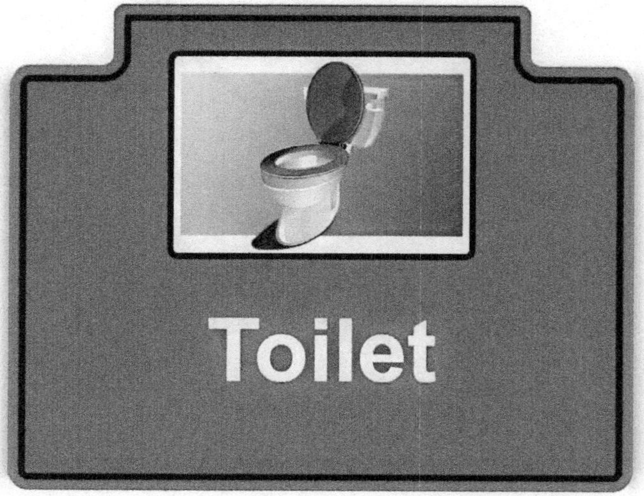

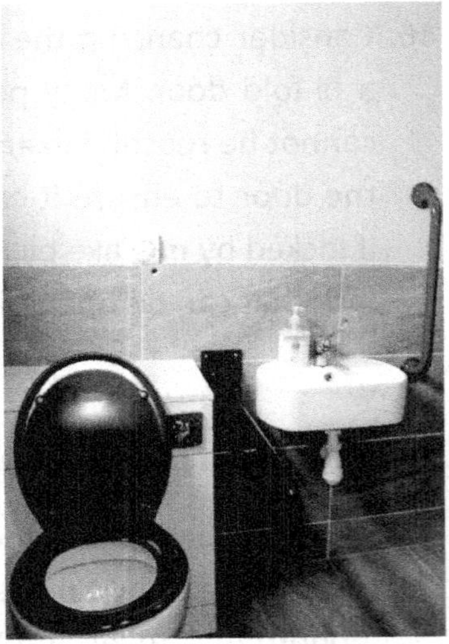

48. Replace the toilet seat with a coloured one to make it easier to see. Toilet seats in colours that contrast with the toilet and with other nearby surfaces can help make these more visible and identifiable.

49. Get a raised toilet seat with side handles to make sitting and getting up easier, such as those found at www.nrshealthcare.co.uk

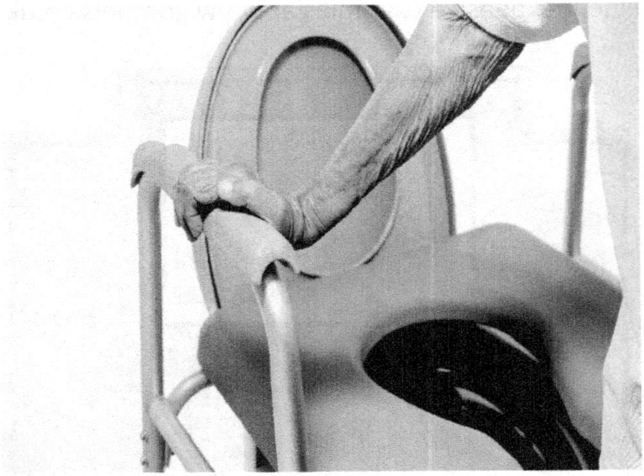

50. Soap holders, toilet brush holders, and even bars of soap in a contrasting colour from the surroundings help provide contrast.

51. People with dementia may find mixer taps challenging to understand. Push-button options on both taps and cisterns can also be confusing. A simple 'push to flush' or 'push to turn on' sign can make things easier. Alternatively, traditional crosshead taps, ideally with both labels and colour cues to distinguish hot and cold taps can help.

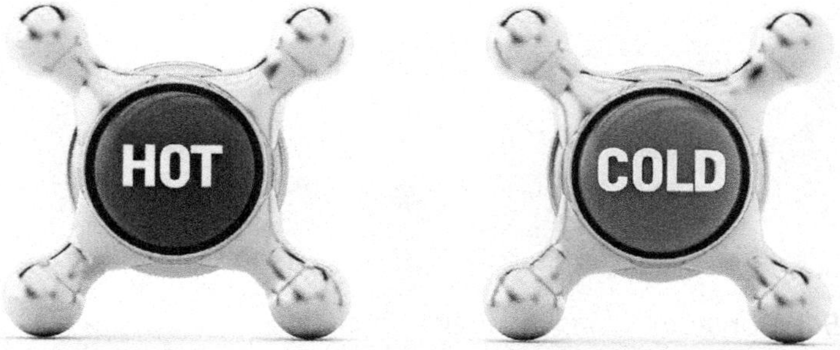

Helpful Tips to Reduce the Risk of Flooding

52. Use a simple notice board or whiteboard near the taps with a message as a reminder, 'Don't Forget to Turn the Tap Off'.

53. Consider using an anti-flood device such as the Magiplug which reduces the risk of scalding and flooding. When an unattended bath or sink reaches a certain depth, the pressure plate opens and releases excess water. The plug also changes colour at 36 degrees centigrade. It can offer a simple and cost-effective way to help prevent

baths and sinks from overflowing. The Magiplug can be found at www.magiplug.com.

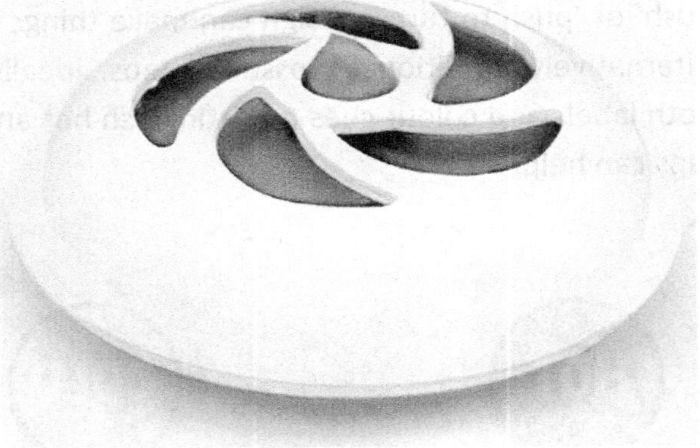

54. Consider using a device such as the 'Blue Fish Alarm', found at www.byretech.com. This device sticks to the side of the bath and when water reaches the chosen height, an alarm sounds to remind the person to turn the tap off.

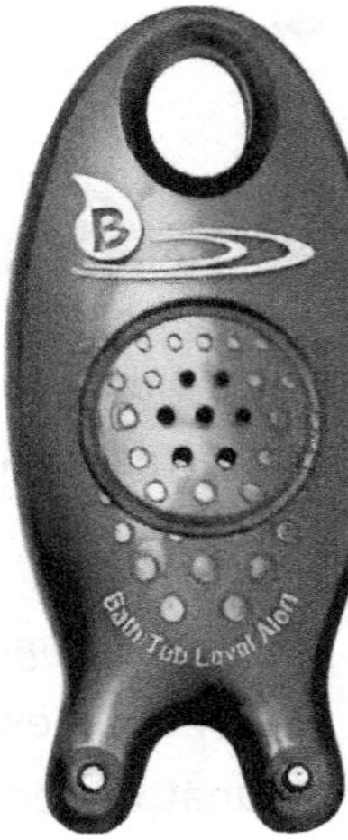

55. Consider a flood detector which can detect an overflow of water on the floor. Once installed in a bathroom or kitchen, the flood detector will immediately alert when a sink or bath overflow occurs. It will also detect water from other sources such as a water leak or burst pipe. These products can be standalone such as those

provided by Ultra Secure or be part of a broader telecare system such as those provided by Tunstall in the UK. In the event of a flood, the system will shut off the water and an alarm will be raised.

Bedroom

Bedrooms are personal spaces for everyone, including people with dementia. Displaying personal items such as photos to personalise the room reminds them it's their space and that they should feel comfortable and relaxed there. Picture albums and family photos also provide excellent conversational prompts and cues.

Sleep is crucial for someone with dementia; disturbed sleep patterns and lack of sleep can lead to increased confusion. If someone is up during the night, the same is the case for other members of the family, leading to all-round disruption in the house and daily life. It's essential to make sure the bedroom is warm and comfortable for a good night's sleep for everyone.

In the bedroom, certain precautions are necessary. Place a bedside lamp, torch, and phone within easy reach of the bed and ensure the area around the bed is free from clutter. Also, make sure that there are no heaters near bedclothes, furniture, or curtains.

A hospital-style bed can be helpful for both you and the person as it can be adjusted to the exact height to make helping someone in and out of bed easier and safer. A commode in the bedroom may also be useful if the person struggles to reach the bathroom. However, depending on the stage of dementia, the person may forget what it's for.

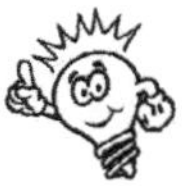

Helpful Tips

56. Paint the trim or the full door in the person's favourite colour. Put a sign with the word 'bedroom' and a photo of a bed on it. This will serve as a reminder, especially during the night with bathroom visits.

57. Being able to recognise the edge of the bed is essential. A bottom bed sheet in a contrasting colour to the top layer and duvet and a different colour again for the carpet helps identify the end of the bed.

58. Consider the use of a bed sensor. If the person gets up and doesn't return within a pre-set time, or if they don't get up in the morning, an alarm is raised. This can be standalone or part of a more extensive telecare system. Several can be found at www.frequencyprecision.com.

59. Consider replacing electric blankets and hot water bottles as the condition progresses, especially if the person becomes incontinent. Microwave heat pads can offer an alternative solution, providing all-night warmth without the risk of scolding.

60. Consider the use of an audio monitor between rooms which will allow you to hear if the person with dementia is out of bed or calling for help.

Outdoors and Garden Area

The feeling of the sun or a pleasant breeze on our skin, the sound of birds chirping, and the rustling of trees blowing in the wind are all things we love. People enjoy being outdoors and those with dementia are no exception.

Decreasing cognitive function often precedes physical decline resulting in many people with dementia still being physically fit and able to enjoy being outdoors. Ensuring the outside area around the house and garden is safe and secure is just as important as the inside living space.

Getting outside can also prove beneficial by giving people with dementia fresh air and vitamin D as well as satisfying a need for contemplation, escape, restoration, and distraction. The combination of sight, smell, and sound offer the potential for critical sensory experiences that help promote well-being.

As most people spend a lot of time during their life outside, it also provides the person with a sense of normality. Designers nowadays in care homes look at the garden as a therapeutic environment, offering an opportunity for physical and mental engagement. The same opportunity exists at home.

The outdoors can offer a different perspective on life. It's a quiet place to sit, often hard to find inside. On a beautiful warm day, a garden can provide a place for activity, socialising, and sensory stimulation.

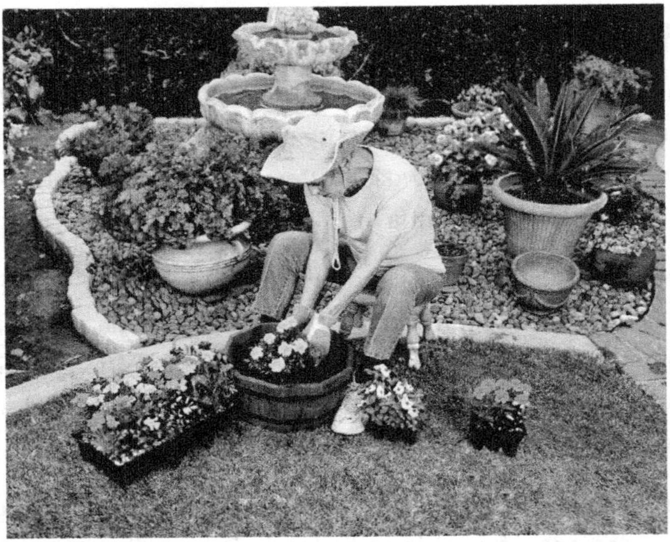

The design of the outdoor space should correlate in many ways to the inside. Keep in mind the need for safe physical accessibility while carefully considering the therapeutic elements of leading a dementia-aware lifestyle.

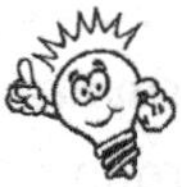

Helpful Tips

61. Ensure the area outside is obstacle and hazard-free, well-lit with night-time security lights.

62. Ensure steps and stairs have handrails. Distractions while negotiating steps such as potted plants should be removed. Installing a sign such as 'Watch Your Step' will act as a simple additional reminder.

63. Painting steps a bright contrasting colour on the trim can help make it easy to see each step.

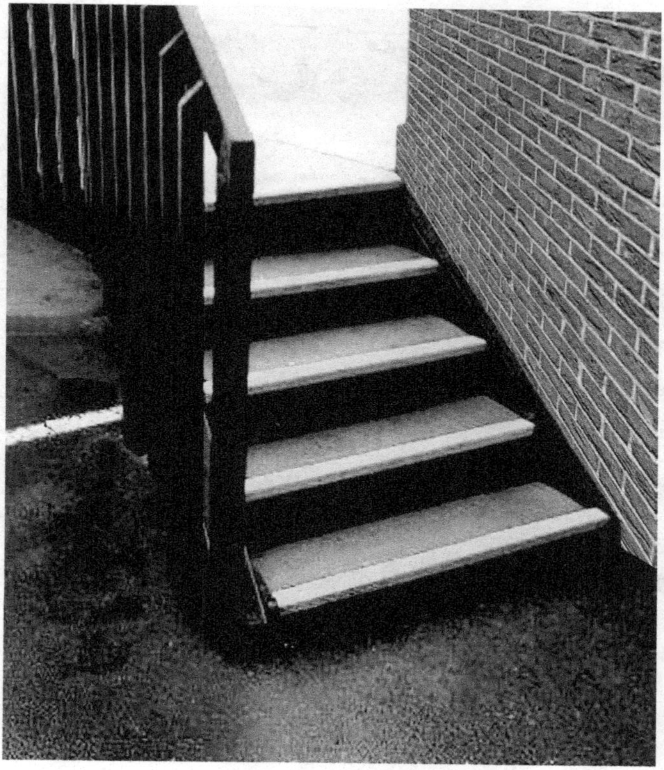

From my personal experience, rubber grips like the ones in the picture below are safer on wet and slippy surfaces but are not entirely dementia-friendly. On one occasion, whilst out walking with my mum, she bent down to pick up what she thought were round coloured coins lying on the ground. It was on a pedestrian crossing, so not a pleasant or safe experience.

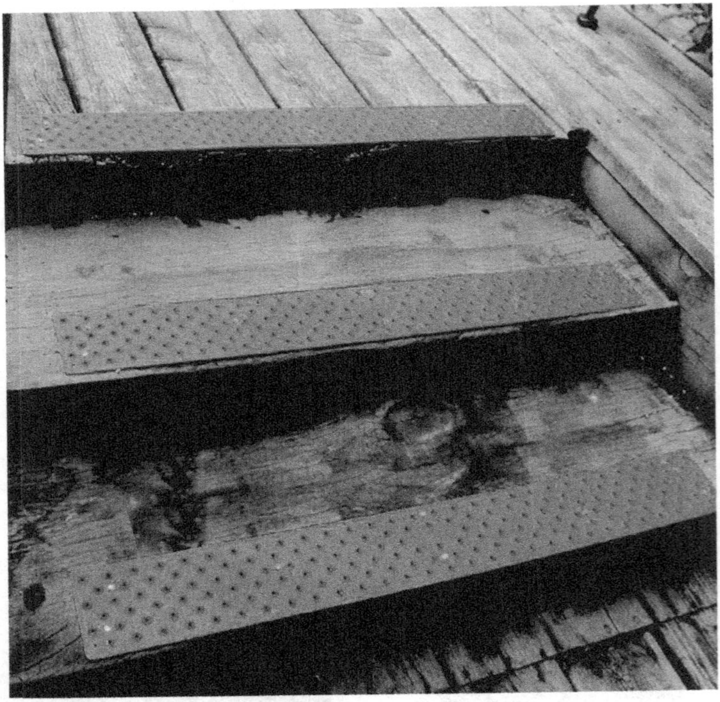

64. Lock away all garden tools, equipment, and poisonous chemicals such as paint, fertilisers, and fuel for a lawnmower.

65. All sets of keys to any motorised vehicles should be secure and inaccessible.

66. If your family member enjoys gardening, raised flower beds allow them to continue to manage the garden. Bamboo or bushes that rustle can provide wonderful stimulation.

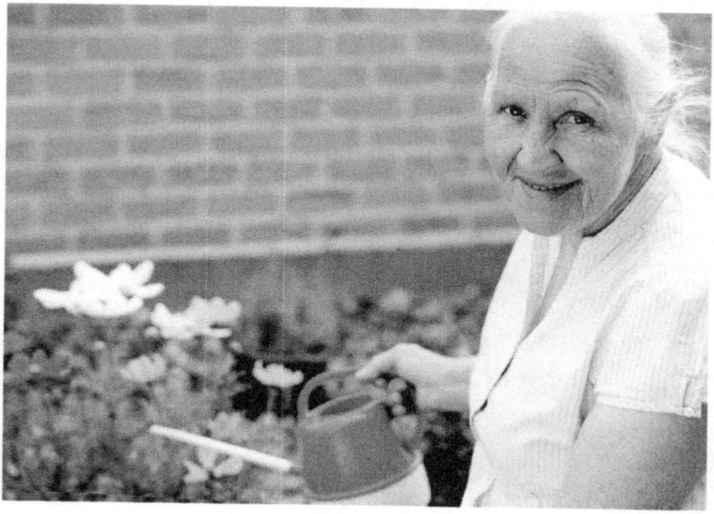

67. Having a focal point in the garden such as a birdbath, water feature, or decorative planter can promote positive stimulation through colour, touch, or smell whilst offering the opportunity to spark memories and encourage conversation.

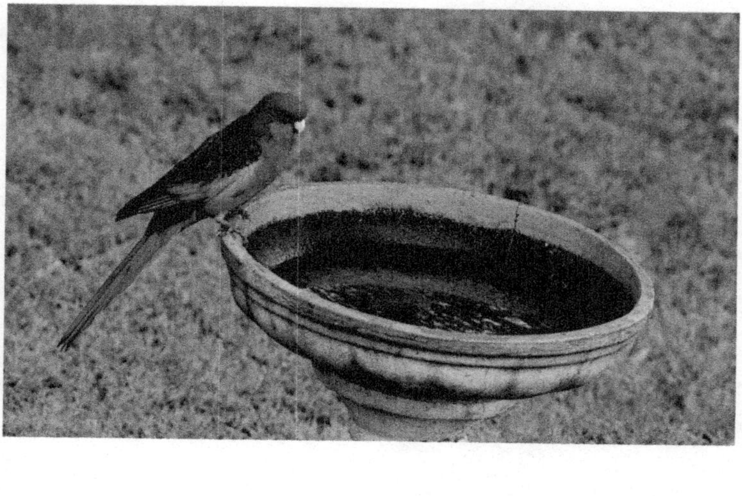

CHAPTER 4

Benefitting from Assistive Technology

Widespread internet coverage is making technology more accessible to everyone and that includes people with dementia and their families. Technological tools are increasingly providing opportunities to live better at home by helping people with dementia improve their well-being, social participation, confidence as well as increase safety and help with potential risks in and outside of the home.

According to www.vodg.org.uk, assistive technology (AT) includes any device or system that allows individuals to perform tasks they would otherwise be unable to do or at least increases the ease and safety with which they are carried out. Solutions can range in complexity from DIY adaptations at home to simple 'low-tech' items, to more 'high-tech' and sophisticated Telecare systems.

Accessing Knowledge and Support

Digital tools can help family carers save time on everyday tasks such as online banking, shopping, booking medical practitioner appointments, and ordering medication. Online support networks and local groups can also prove helpful. The internet opens up a world of care-giving training, web-based blogs, and platforms to facilitate and improve knowledge and support.

More and more people with dementia such as Kate Swaffer and Wendy Mitchell have used online blogs to share their experience of living with dementia. Dementia Diaries in the UK is another great platform that brings together people's diverse experiences of living with dementia through a series of audio diaries. It can help someone with dementia feel more in control, informed, and connected to a wider network of people in the same situation. My own blog can be found at www.clickdementia.com.

Participating in Enjoyable Activities

The internet is also increasingly being used to provide activities for people with dementia such as online puzzles, games, and music. YouTube can be used as a reminiscence tool to engage people with their hobbies and memories of people and places.

Video games designed for cognitive and physical stimulation, especially in the early stages of dementia, are becoming increasingly available. Websites such as www.lumosity.com

have brain training apps that provide interactive ways to improve memory, increase focus, and find calm.

Finally, Skype is a great tool to keep in touch with family and friends both home and abroad.

Overcoming Obstacles

Many people with dementia have a lack of interest and motivation to learn about the internet and technology. This is usually based on the stage of dementia or a lack of confidence and fear of doing things wrong. It can be difficult for people with dementia to overcome but if they have used any form of device before their diagnosis (e.g. a tablet or desktop computer) this may be the way forward.

If you need help, courses such as "Learn my way" provide instructions on how to use the internet. It also provides links to information on a range of health conditions including dementia.

Getting the Balance Right

Of course, AT should never take the place of personal care at home. It's important to remember too that what works for one person may not for another. A voice coming from a prompt in the corner of the room may be confusing and frightening rather than reassuring for some. Accidental triggering of alarms can also leave the person fearful of technology.

Utilising Telecare

Telecare offers elderly people living in their own home the opportunity to access support or response services when needed. When family members are out working, knowing that someone at home with dementia is safe is essential for peace of mind and for enabling other family members to get on with life. This type of support is particularly helpful for people living alone with dementia.

Telecare systems can include community alarms, sensors, movement detectors, and video conferencing. Examples include fall alarms, safety sensors for risks such as gas leaks and bath floods, changes in temperature and activity monitors. In the event of extreme temperatures, sensors will send a warning signal if the temperature is very low, very high or changes suddenly. This can be particularly beneficial if a pan has been left on the stove or if the temperature in a room is so low that it could have the potential to cause hypothermia. A sensor can also be placed on a bed or chair and alerted if the person doesn't return in a pre-set time.

These devices communicate with each other via a hub connected to a phone line or the internet and are activated in the event of the relevant trigger. An alarm will be raised with a central monitoring service, which in turn can:

- Talk to the person through an intercom
- Contact a carer or someone in the family if they live nearby

- Contact another professional who can help
- Contact emergency services

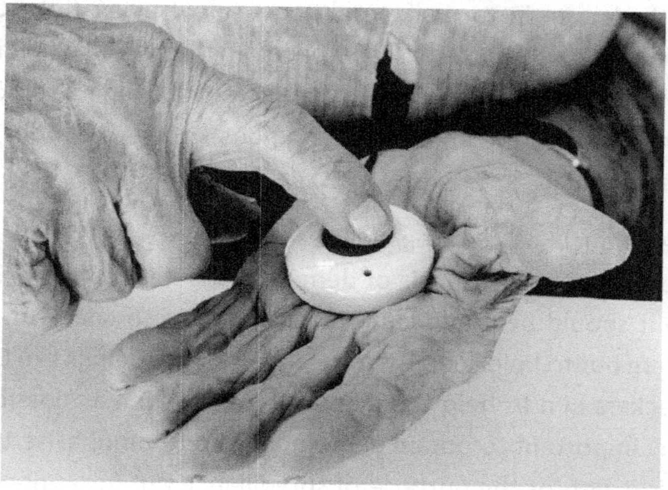

The connected services can also be checked remotely if the person with dementia switches it off.

More advanced 'intelligent' systems are designed to recognise changes in activity levels such as visits to the toilet which may indicate that a person's condition is deteriorating. Data transmitted via Telecare systems allows us to understand what's going on. For example, when the kettle gets turned on, we know the person is up during the day.

Services can be customised to address the individual needs of each person and their caregivers for memory support, helping with daily activities, maintaining social contact, and increased safety.

Getting Outdoors

Solutions are also being developed to support people with dementia to walk freely and safely away from the home, reducing the risk of becoming lost and allowing communication between the family member and a remote family carer to help if something goes wrong or simply for reassurance.

Items such as tracking devices can help with safety. A person with a diagnosis of dementia still has human rights so it should be made clear that this is not to check up on them but to help keep them safe and sound. Things like GPS trackers aim to help the person to live as well as possible. It is important to obtain agreement and to emphasise that this is not for the purpose of surveillance but for improved quality of life.

Looking Ahead to Technology of the Future

According to recent research, socially assistive robots offer promising solutions to assist with communication, reducing isolation and disconnection from communities as well as supporting daily activities. This type of technology obviously raises ethical issues and the need to remember that nothing can replace human social interaction. Although research in this field is still in its early stages, studies have shown favourable results among participants with dementia. An example can be found at www.cutii.io/en/.

Helpful Tips

68. Make use of several DIY or 'low-tech' ways to assist people with dementia to overcome memory problems. Well-positioned reminder boards or notices in key areas of the house can alleviate distress. Simple things such as post-it pads, a whiteboard, or a calendar provide an easy and cost-effective solution to memory prompts and reminders in mild stage dementia. Something as simple as chimes hanging inside the front door will raise an alert that the front door has been opened.

69. Make use of the 'stand-alone' technological solutions that exist today on the market including calendar clocks, memo clocks, locator devices, medication prompts, memo minders and picture telephones. A range of helpful devices can be found online.

70. Standalone automated prompts and reminders can also help to stay safe around the home. These can be motion or time activated.

71. Make enquiries to find out if community telecare services are available in your area. Many government bodies now offer free or fee-based telecare services. In countries such as the UK, the local Fire and Rescue Service offer a free Fire Safety inspection for all elderly or vulnerable adults living at home. Many government strategies are also in place offering free community alarm services and other associated telecare add-ons such as remote smoke, fire, carbon monoxide, and flood detection. Private companies such as Canary Care, Chubb, Tunstall, and Tynetec in the UK offer a range of similar services.

72. Installing a wireless two-way home camera will allow you to keep an eye at home whilst out or talk to each other for re-assurance or if there's a problem. Again, this shouldn't be to spy on the person from afar but to offer a workable solution to providing help at home in the event of a problem.

73. Here are a few tools that might work well for you and your family:

- Tablets such as My Home Helper
- Gadgets such as Amazon Echo and Alexa.
- Apps such as Jointly
- Plug-ins to connect through a TV as found at www.heyherbie.com and www.independa.com.
- Devices to stay connected such as those at www.sociavi.com and www.konnekt.com.au.
- Home monitoring and communication devices such as this found at www.grandcare.com.

CHAPTER 5

Staying Close to Home

Enjoying Safer Walking

People with dementia still enjoy walking outdoors and it offers so many physical and psychological benefits. Spending regular time out in the daylight will help to set the body clock and establish a natural rhythm for the day, promoting better sleep and reduced stress.

Having to stop driving can be upsetting for someone with dementia, so it's essential to find alternative means of staying connected to the local community and neighbourhood. Family trips to the supermarket help maintain a sense of worth as an ongoing contributor to the household.

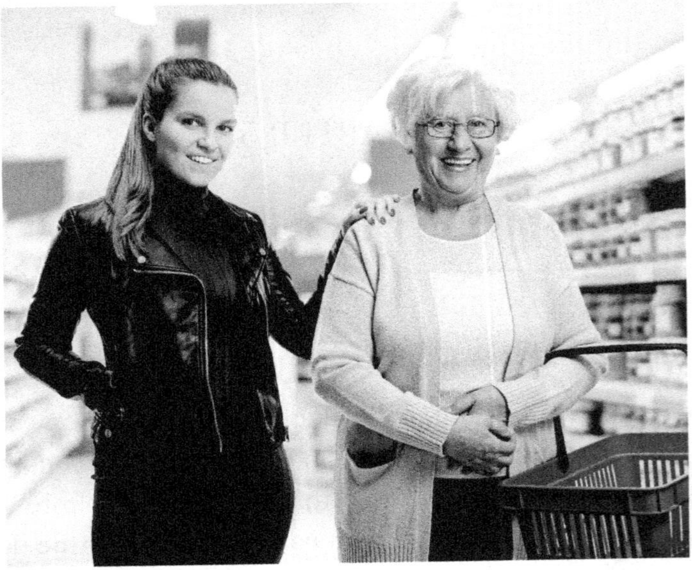

An ongoing concern, however, for family carers is the person coming to harm, especially if they want to leave the house for a walk on their own. By introducing some of the practical steps below, you can help the person enjoy a degree of freedom in a safer way, whilst alleviating your own concerns.

Helpful Tips

74. Purchase ID jewellery such as those offered by Medic Alert. If the person becomes lost or hurt, it has a telephone number someone can call for help. Various styles of pendants or bracelets are available and can be found at www.medicalert.org.uk.

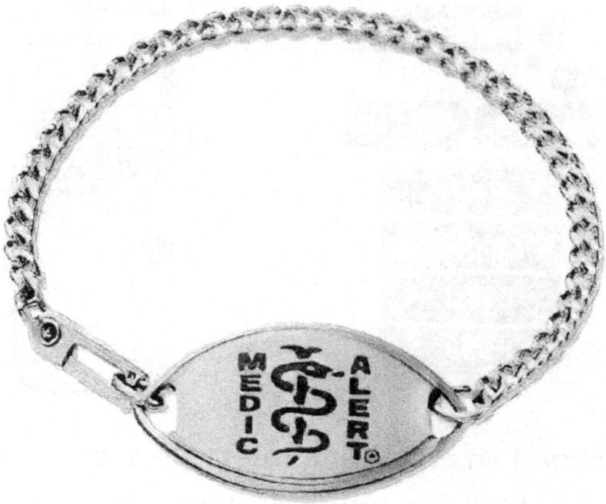

75. Download the Proximity app if out walking together in town or a shopping mall. Wearing a connecting magnetic button, if the person wanders out of range, a notification through a Smartphone immediately alerts the family carer.

76. Mobile phones are useful for contacting help in an emergency. Phones with features like larger buttons, easier to see screens, and buttons that can be programmed to call someone if lost are great options. Examples include the Ownfone and the Dora Secure 580.

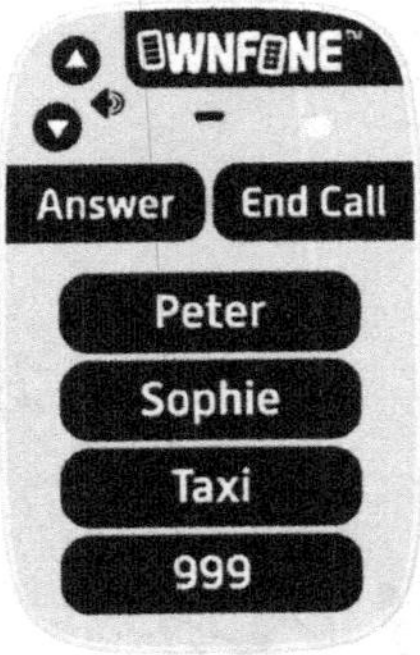

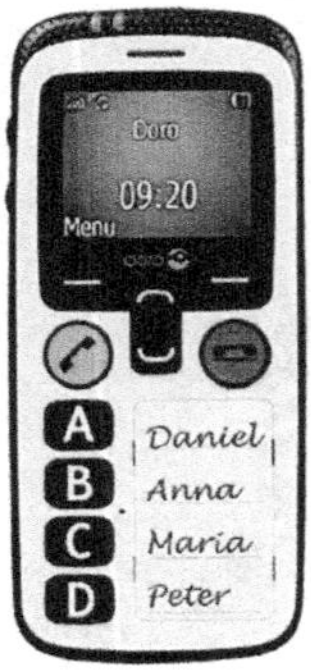

A simplified smart phone interface such as that found at www.baldphone.com can also make life easier.

77. Consider using a personal alarm. Many are directly linked via telephone to operators who can get assistance to a person in need of help. The Buddi alarm offers a fall sensor as an additional feature.

78. Consider using a GPS tracking watch with mobile. These devices send alerts as soon as someone leaves the house or a specific area or wanders into a zone pre-programmed as a no-go area. Many offer two-way calling with an automatic answering, loudspeaker and SOS call facility. Watches such as those by Tech Silver in the UK will go through a list of contacts automatically until someone answers. Other examples include the Watchu Guardian and Yepzon.

79. Alternatively, consider GPS Smart shoes. Built into the shoe itself, the device cannot be seen but enables you to follow someone's footsteps from your computer or Smartphone. Examples can be found at www.techsilver.co.uk.

Preventing Leaving Home Unexpectedly and Getting Lost

One of the main problems for someone living with dementia is not only the harm that may occur at home but also the fact that they may wander away from home unexpectedly and become lost or injured. But there is a lot nowadays that can be done to help.

The dictionary definition of the word wander is "to walk or move aimlessly". In dementia, however, wandering often has a purpose, whether caused by an underlying physical problem such as being in pain, thirsty or hungry; feeling stressful and agitated; wanting to go 'home'; or seeking out something or someone from the past. Wandering can take place at any time of day but is particularly dangerous at night.

Prevention is better than cure so understanding the cause of wandering will help. Satisfying simple physical unmet needs, having a daily routine, remaining involved in activities, and getting outdoors regularly whether going to the shops or gardening can help.

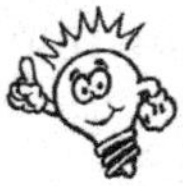

Helpful Tips

80. Put a sign on the front door that says something like 'We are Staying Home Today'.

81. Put away all daytime clothes at night to avoid prompting the person to get up and get dressed in the middle of the night. Briefcases, suitcases, shoes at the door, car

keys, hats on the hat-rack, and other visible reminders of travelling that may remind the person of leaving can also be removed.

82. Hang a clock in the bedroom to help the person make sense of what time of day it is. This will help the person refrain from getting out of bed thinking it's daytime. Some dementia-specific clocks show the time as a.m. or p.m. Others use a 24-hour clock. Examples can be found at www.shop.alzheimers.org.uk or www.dementia.livebetterwith.org.

83. Place a floor pressure mat inside the front door that sounds an alarm if stood on – this will let you know someone is possibly leaving the house.

84. Consider the use of a motion-activated voice player such as those by Tech Silver in the UK which plays a pre-recorded message when movement is detected.

85. Use devices that signal when a door or window is open. This can be as simple as a bell or wind-chime or as sophisticated as a sensor alarm that sounds if the front door is opened and a message transmitted through to the family carer or monitoring centre. This can be fine-tuned to specific times such as night-time.

86. Consider telecare systems that can also automatically transmit live video to the mobile of a family member when the front door sensors are activated by the door opening.

Being Prepared for an Emergency

Of course, we can't guarantee that a family member with dementia won't leave home unexpectedly, so it's important to be prepared.

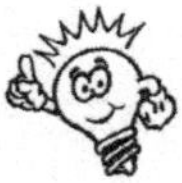

Helpful Tips

87. Label personal items such as wallet, purse, and shoes with details and a contact number.

88. Build up a network of friendly neighbours, friends and family who can all support the person if found out alone and in distress.

89. Check if your local area offers a service such as those below that aim to quickly identify any person who appears lost and confused:

    - Purple Alert (Scotland, UK)
    - The Herbert Protocol (England, UK)
    - Safe Return (Australia)
    - Silver Alert (USA)

CHAPTER 6

Stopping Doorstep Crime, Scams & Fraud

Bogus callers and rogue traders purposefully target older people, seeing them as vulnerable and easy to steal from. 53% of people aged 65+ in the UK have been targeted by bogus callers – the average age of a scam victim being 75 years old. People with dementia are particularly at risk, especially those living alone.

All too often, older people fall prey to doorstep crime daily, often referred to as 'knock knock' burglary. From bogus callers to rogue traders, doorstep criminals are cunning, creative, and very convincing. Anyone can be fooled as these people are professional con-artists. However, older people and especially those with dementia are particularly vulnerable.

Bogus Callers

These people try to get into the home or obtain personal details by pretending to be someone they're not, including government staff, charity collectors, meter readers, and police officers. In reality, they are nothing more than lowdown criminals trying to steal money and personal valuables.

Rogue Traders

Rogue traders usually cold-call. They offer to carry out work on the house or driveway. In reality, they charge inflated prices for shoddy or unnecessary work. They will often say the work is urgent and needs to be carried out immediately. They will ask for payment upfront and even offer to drive the person to the bank if they don't have the cash at home.

Many rogue traders pose as gardeners or companies offering 'free surveys' to find out if you need work carried out such as wall coatings. They offer to do work but say they need to check something in the home first, which is when they search the house for items or cash.

These criminals often work in pairs. One may ask you to come around to the back of the house to highlight a 'bogus' repair that needs urgent attention. Meanwhile, the other slips into the house to look around for something to steal – a practice known as distraction burglary.

Reputable companies are keen to advertise their services and happily display their name on the van. But rogue traders often have no writing on their vans. Another clue (but not always the case) is the front dashboard of the van. Regular 'working' vans are packed with brochures, post, ID pads, receipts, etc. – rogue traders often won't have this material.

All callers should offer ID. In the UK, it's illegal for a company to cold-call unless they have registered with the police. Often, rogue traders will say that they have left their badge at home today.

These unscrupulous criminals are experts in their craft, very convincing, and highly plausible.

Postal and Email Fraud

This includes lottery or prize scams where people are told they have won a massive amount of money and all they have to do is send a fee to release it. Scammers also send out official-looking letters from banks and building societies asking for personal details. Another favourite is a letter or email from the government offering a tax rebate. There are also catalogues selling a variety of products, guaranteeing prizes for those who order, often followed up by a phone call confirming the 'win' or being told to look out for further letters in the post.

Investment scams, get rich quick schemes, and miracle cures are all common ways of scamming money from unsuspecting citizens.

Parcel Delivery Scams

These involve cards being put through the door stating that a parcel was to be delivered, but no-one was home. It comes with a premium rate phone number that turns out to be a long, recorded message, incurring a hefty phone bill.

Scammers are professionals in their field and make their scams look authentic. Using words such as 'guaranteed prize', 'unclaimed prize', 'time is running out', 'claim your prize now', they can very quickly hook their victims.

False testimonials, photos of 'previous winners', false authoritative names and titles all add to the false picture they create.

Scammers even build very impressive websites to where they refer the person in an attempt to verify their 'company'. The victim becomes excited and begins to focus on the 'prize' rather than the fact that they are being asked to send cash to claim it.

Some countries offer services to stop junk mail but the reality is that mailing companies have a legal obligation to deliver all addressed mail.

Telephone Scams

Cold-callers make contact by telephone, claiming to be from investment companies and will offer to sell investments that, according to them, offer huge financial gain. But these are worthless or don't even exist.

In countries such as the UK, the aim of registering with the 'Telephone Preference Service' is to stop unsolicited telephone calls. But in reality, many nuisance calls still get through.

Many elderly people are too embarrassed to report the crime or cannot even remember the offence taking place. Even if they do, the prosecution against the perpetrator becomes extremely difficult as people with dementia are viewed as 'unreliable' witnesses. There is often little that the police or trading standards can do and the culprits get away scot-free to strike again, all too aware that the group they target is unable to put up any kind of defence.

Meanwhile, elderly victims of crime deteriorate in health faster than non-victims – savings accumulated over a lifetime lost. Families are left to pick up the pieces, stressed at how they could have 'allowed' such a thing to happen, hurt for their relatives, enraged at the fact that their hands are tied in ensuring the culprits are brought to justice.

The aim is to prevent scams rather than deal with the consequences after the fact. There are many precautions we can guide older relatives to take when presented with a stranger at the door – the simplest being to use a nearby window before answering. Then only allowing callers in if they have an appointment and their identity card has been confirmed by calling the company to ensure authenticity. The caller can also be asked to call back at another time when a family member is there. We can also encourage them when in any doubt at all, to refrain from answering the door.

However, this is not the situation with people with dementia. Especially for those living alone; strangers can be seen as friends who will more often than not be invited into the house. When the person is lonely, any friendly face at all is a new friend to be welcomed. The crime can also be forgotten by the victim very quickly.

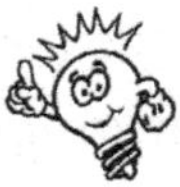

Helpful Tips

90. Ensure all valuables are placed in a secure place.

91. Display a 'No Cold Calling' card in the window. However, unfortunately, this can also give the criminal a clue that an elderly person is living in the house, as can railings and wheelchair ramps.

92. Be aware of increased calls from strangers. Continually look for warning signs – flyers, unusual amounts of post, large cash withdrawals. Monitor increased use of cheque books, envelopes, and stamps.

93. Talk to neighbours and ask them to watch out for strangers or strange vans parked outside or on the driveway.

94. Building a trusted traders list based on recommendations from family and friends can also help.

95. Consider asking the person to sign up with a credit reference company and checking this together on a regular basis for any unusual activity.

96. Arrange for the telephone number to be ex-directory.

97. Ensure the phone cannot accept withheld numbers.

98. Use a call blocking device such as the Truecall Call Blocker or check to see if the phone has a call blocking facility. Block all numbers other than those on a trusted list. Call

blockers screen incoming phone calls and either block any unknown or unauthorised numbers or transfer them to a nominated family member or guardian. Telecalm also offers call blocking and screening facility. It can be found at www.telecalmprotects.com.

99. Consider re-directing mail to a trusted family member.

100. Install a real or dummy security camera with a sticker saying, ‘Smile. You are on camera’.

101. Install a video doorbell which allows you to see and speak to someone at the door from your phone, tablet, or PC. Those offered by Ring are popular examples. Alternatively, products such as the ‘Victure security outdoor camera 1080p’ allows motion-detected viewing and communication with welcome (or unwelcome) guests at the front door.

Final Words

Before you go, I would like to thank you for purchasing my book and reading it to the end.

Implementing all of the steps listed in this book may seem like an overwhelming task, but it's important to remember that not all of them are necessary at once. Some of the suggestions above may not be suitable for everyone – some may be relevant, others not, while others may require tweaks here and there.

Family carers are becoming increasingly informed and empowered in seeking out or fine-tuning solutions to suit their particular situation, environment, and the person they care for. When my mother was first diagnosed, we had already shared a lifetime together, giving me a head start on understanding her way of thinking, feelings, ideas as well as areas of potential vulnerability. It was a case of taking one day at a time, building knowledge as I went – experience becoming my best teacher.

Creating a safe and dementia-aware home proved mutually beneficial – the well-being of my mother resulting in increased feelings of well-being in me.

If you have found this book helpful, please provide an online review. This will allow me to continue to write books that are relevant for people living well at home with dementia.

I am always looking for ways to improve what I do and I would love to hear from you at cath@clickdementia.com.

About the Author

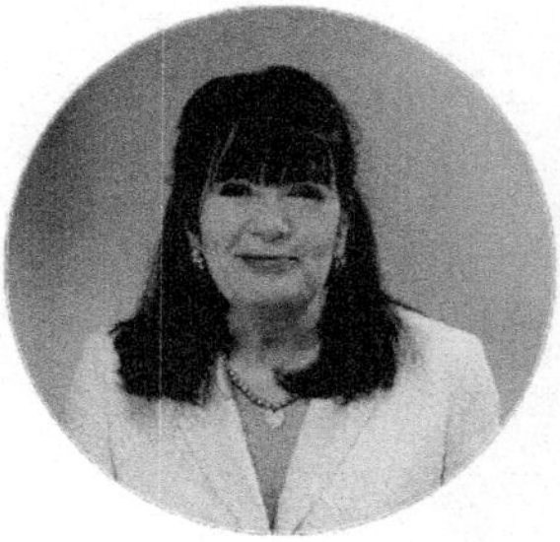

Catherine Verner is an experienced family caregiver spanning a decade, an MSc graduate in Dementia Studies, writer and blogger.

With a decade of practical experience as a family carer, coupled with formal training, she has developed an in-depth and insightful understanding of pre/post-diagnosis and advanced stage dementia, the everyday challenges faced, as well as creative ways in which to support these and promote well-being in both the individual and the family.

Passionate about using her skills and experience to support others, she is in the process of using her knowledge of cutting-edge theory, innovative approaches to care, and research in the field of dementia to create a series of books aimed at supporting those living at home in the community.

Dementia Care at Home Series

Other Books in this Series

Dementia Caregiver: With You. For You. About You.

Inspirational Messages of Support for Dementia Family Caregivers Everywhere

When someone you care about is diagnosed with Alzheimer's disease or another form of dementia, the future can suddenly seem daunting. Stress may overwhelm you and spill into your relationships, work, and family life.

This book of carefully compiled inspirational images and messages by an experienced caregiver offers a touching and refreshing approach to providing dementia care at home.

Join the author for an enriching, heartfelt journey of motivation and empowerment as you learn to:

- Nurture the positive aspects of your care-giving role
- Expand into your role in a holistic way
- Embrace positive and insightful information about dementia
- Take care of yourself as a caregiver

A beautiful blend of inspiration, reflection and recognition – allow this book to connect with the caregiver within. Invest in yourself by bringing this delightful ray of light into your life.

Made in the USA
Monee, IL
04 November 2026

67384402R00056